He's Not Dead Yet

by Amy & Ryan Green
illustrated by Ryan Green

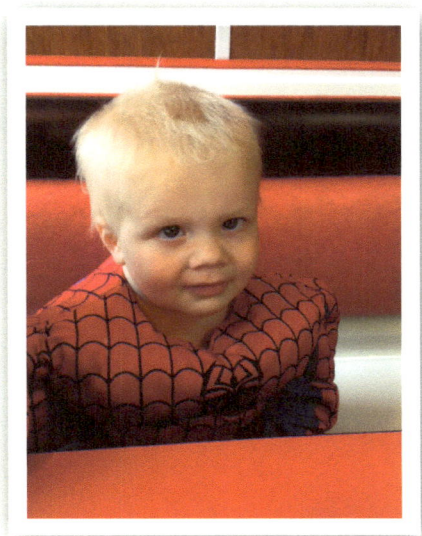

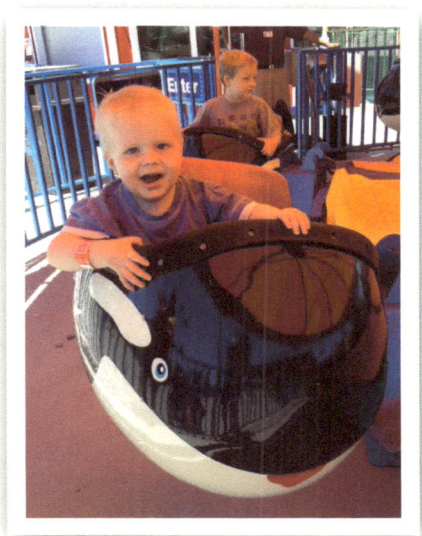

Dedication

Dedicated to our beloved son, Joel Evan Green, who inspired us to write this book. Every day of Joel's life is a miracle and teaches us how to live in the shadow of death and fear no evil. Joel reminds us that we are not dead yet, so we knit our hearts together, focus our eyes on our eternal hope in Christ and keep practicing love, because "if we have a faith that can move mountains, but do not have love, we are nothing." (1 Corinthians 13)

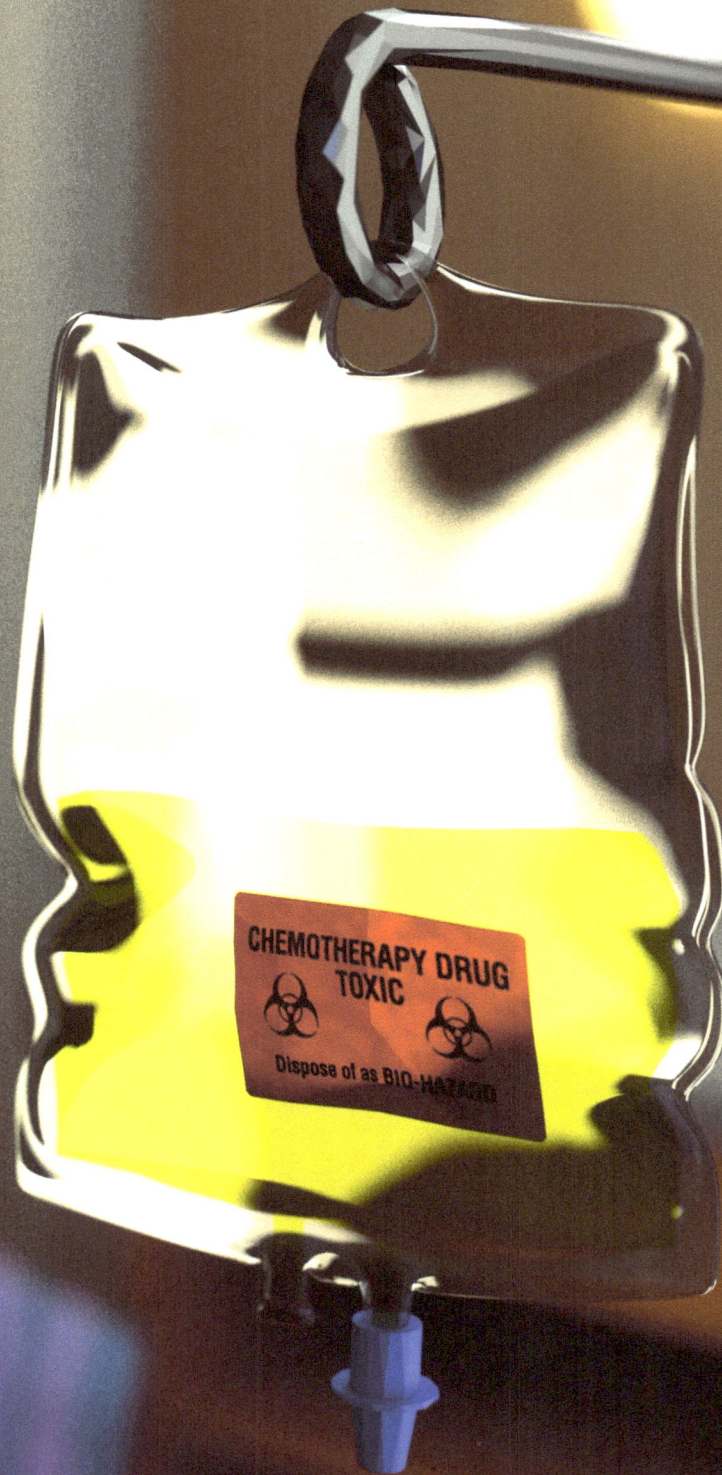

CHEMOTHERAPY DRUG
TOXIC

Dispose of as BIO-HAZARD

My little brother is very sick.

He has a disease the doctors can't fix.

They say the chemo failed and he will die.

My brother doesn't know he's dying.

So he's not sad and he's not crying.

I wish I could be that way too...

because he's not dead yet.

He might not blow out candles on his cake.

What will happen to the wishes he'd make?

I guess there might not be a party this year.

I dream about what I'd like to be.

My brother can't have any dreams.

But maybe we could share just one or two,

since he's not dead yet.

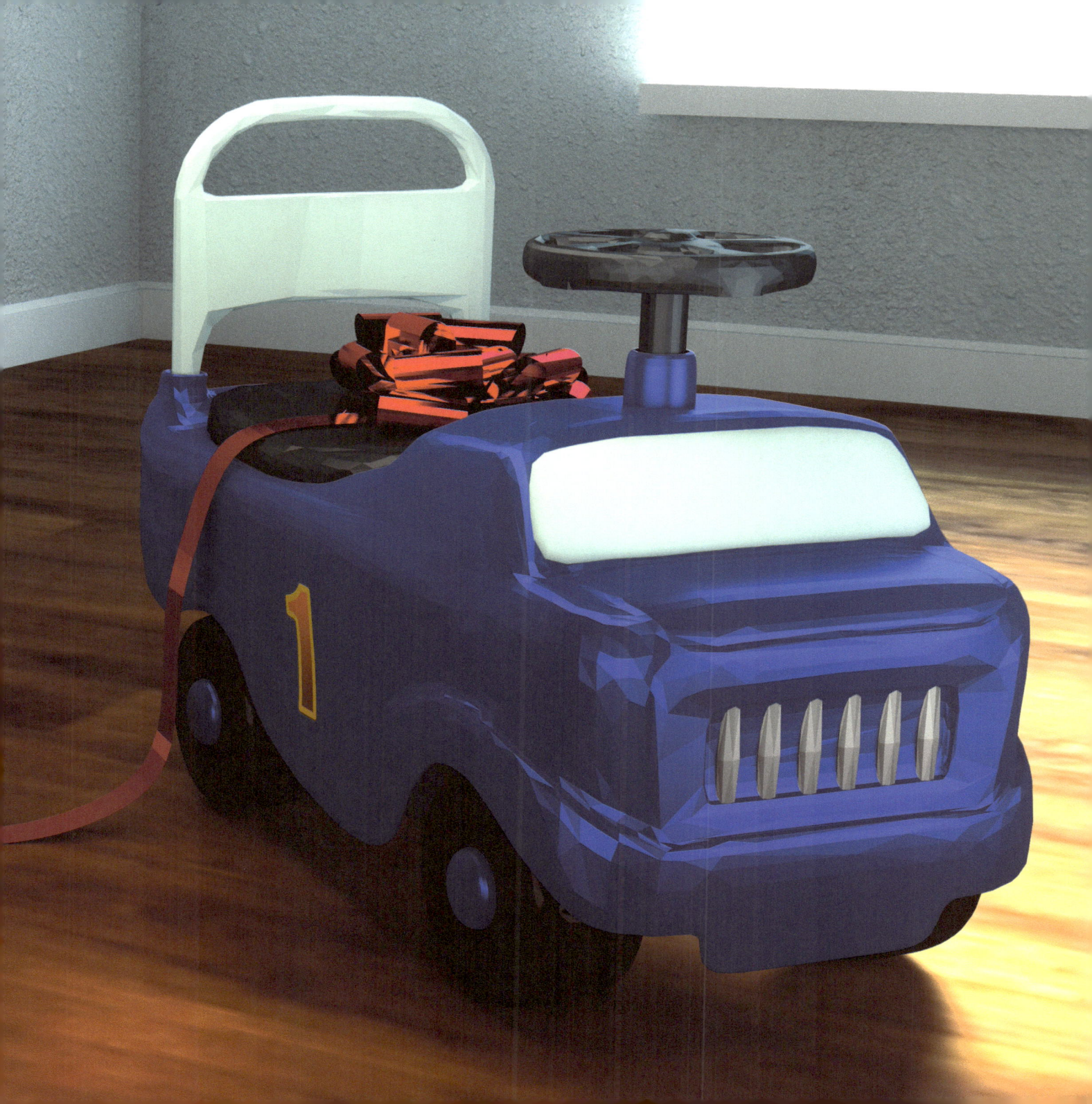

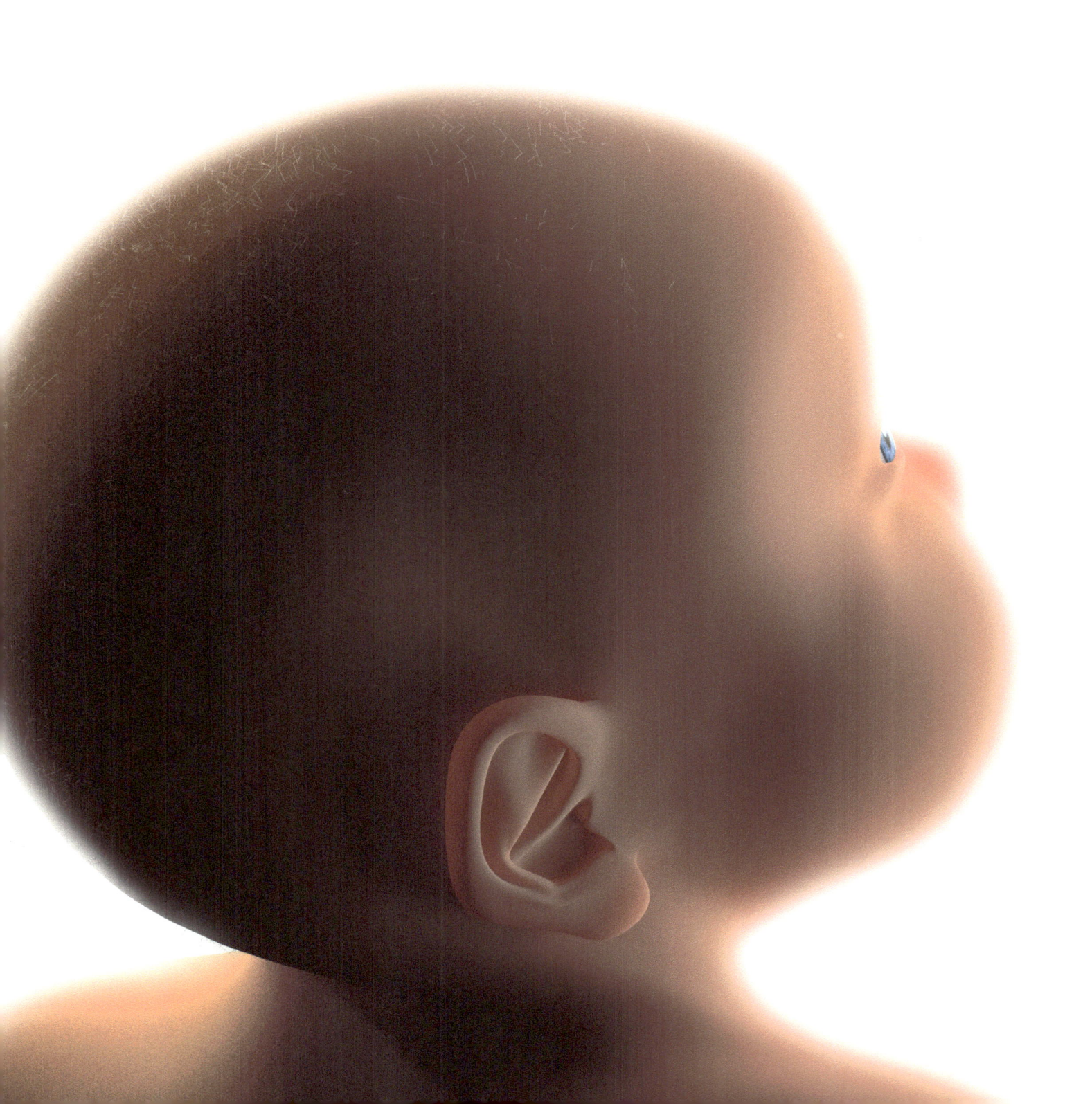

I really don't know what to do.

I don't feel scared, so I'm confused.

My mom calls it "peace" because we pray.

I learned about heaven a little last night.

Dad said it's full of God's bright light.

I bet my brother would love to meet Jesus,

but he's not dead yet.

I pray for a miracle every day.

Because Jesus took our sins away.

He took our sickness, by His wounds we are healed.

There are many plans that we can't plan.

But I can still hold his hand.

And tell him that I love him, you know?

Because he's not dead yet.

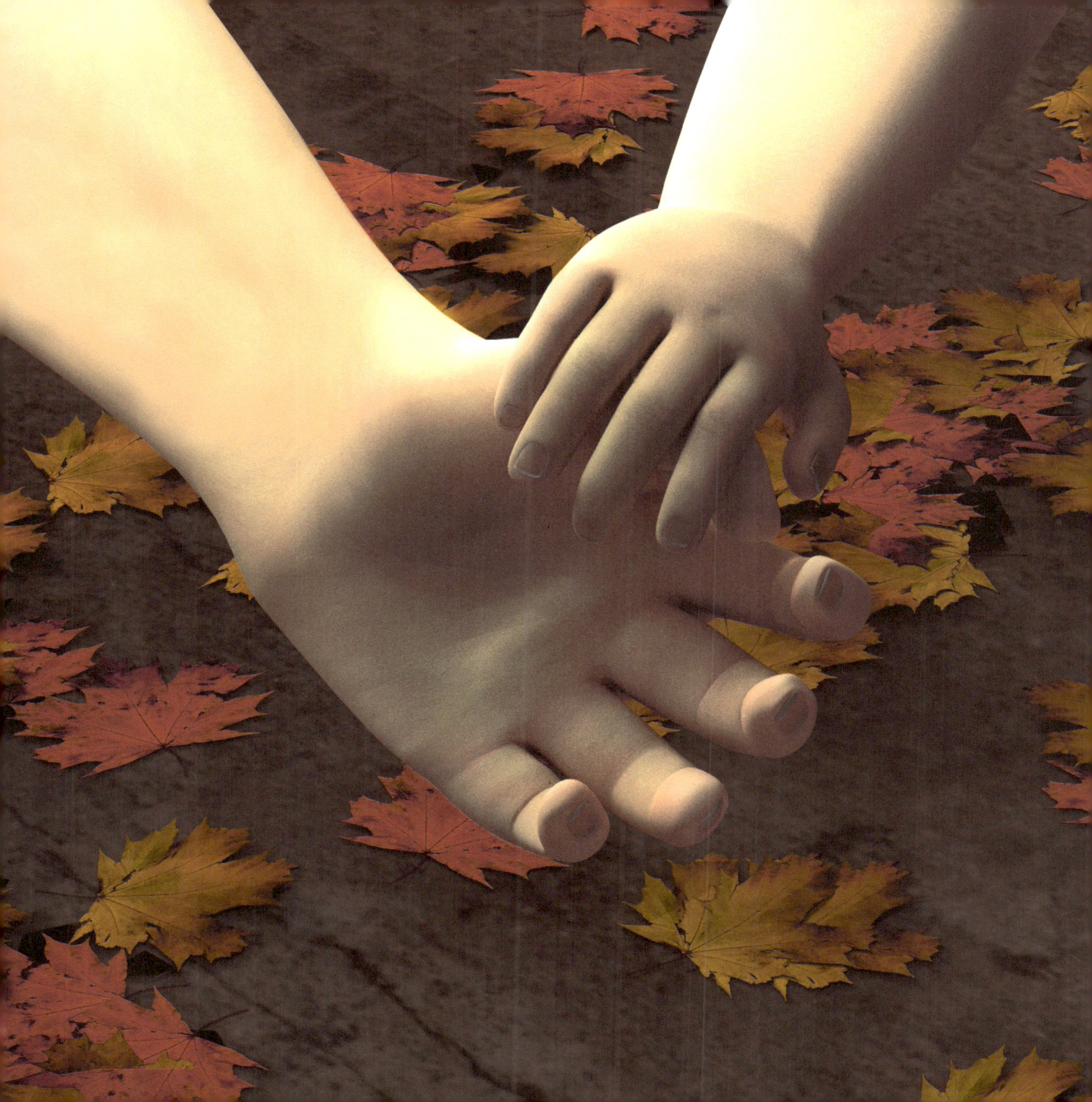

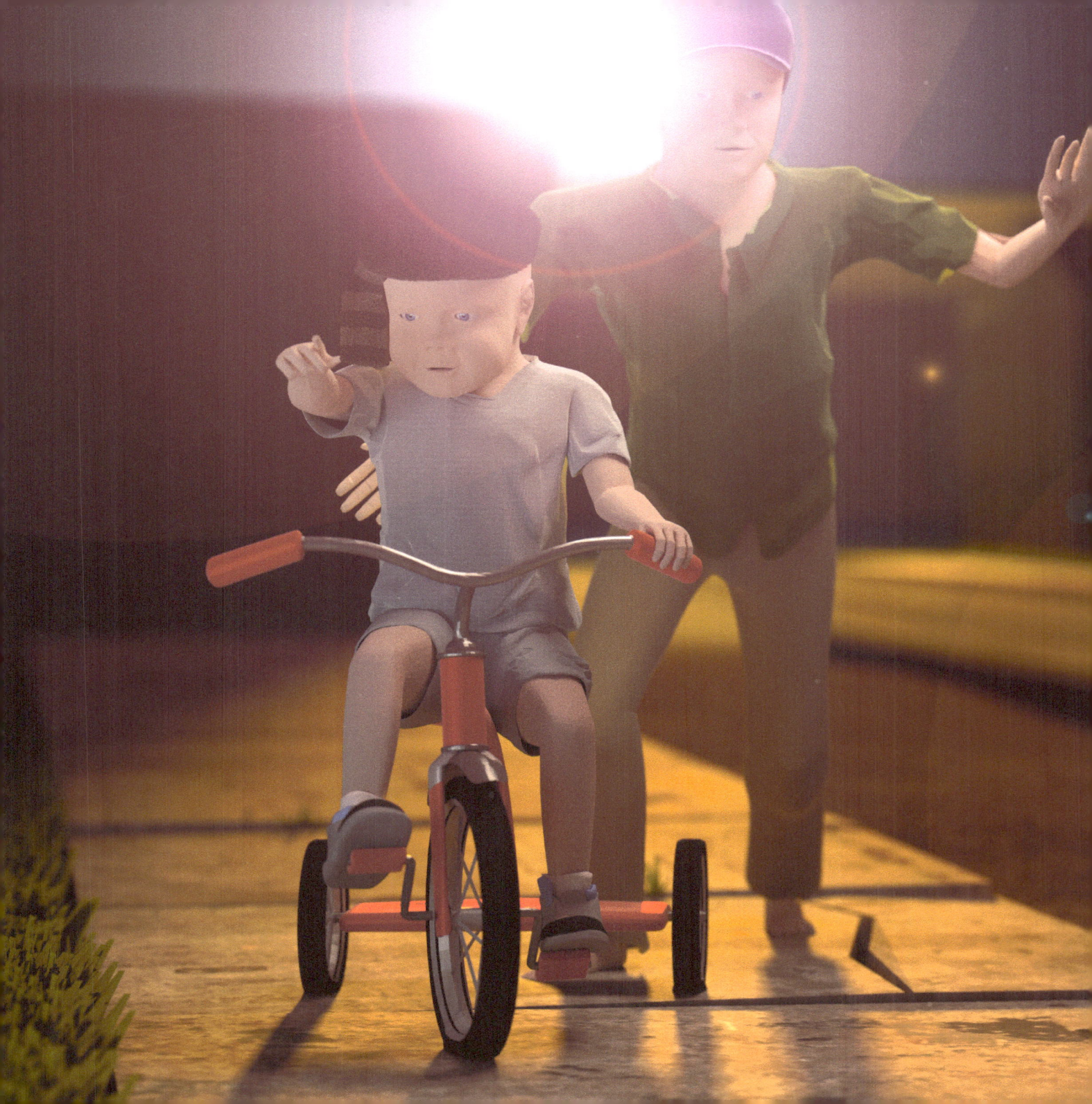

My mom has been taking photographs,

of me and my brothers when we laugh.

I guess there are still some fun times left.

I can sing him songs he likes.

I can push him on his trike.

I'm going to love him, even if I can lose him.

Because he's not dead yet.

Dad went to bed early. Dinner made him cry.

He looked at my brother and his one good eye,

and he knew my brother couldn't eat, only drink.

I wonder what will happen if I love him a bunch,

and he still goes to Heaven; it will hurt so much.

But I'd miss not knowing him while he is here,

and he's not dead yet.

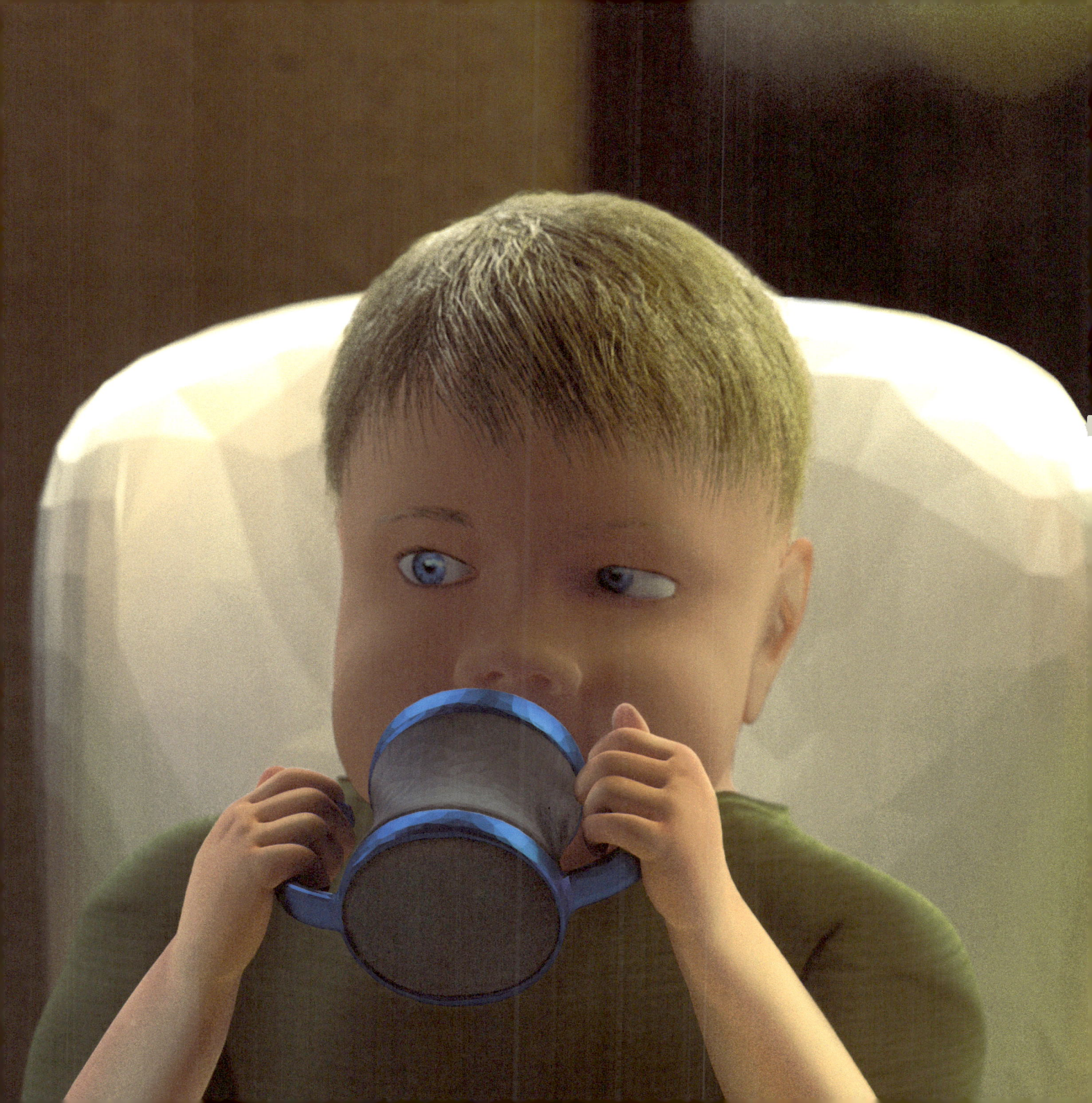

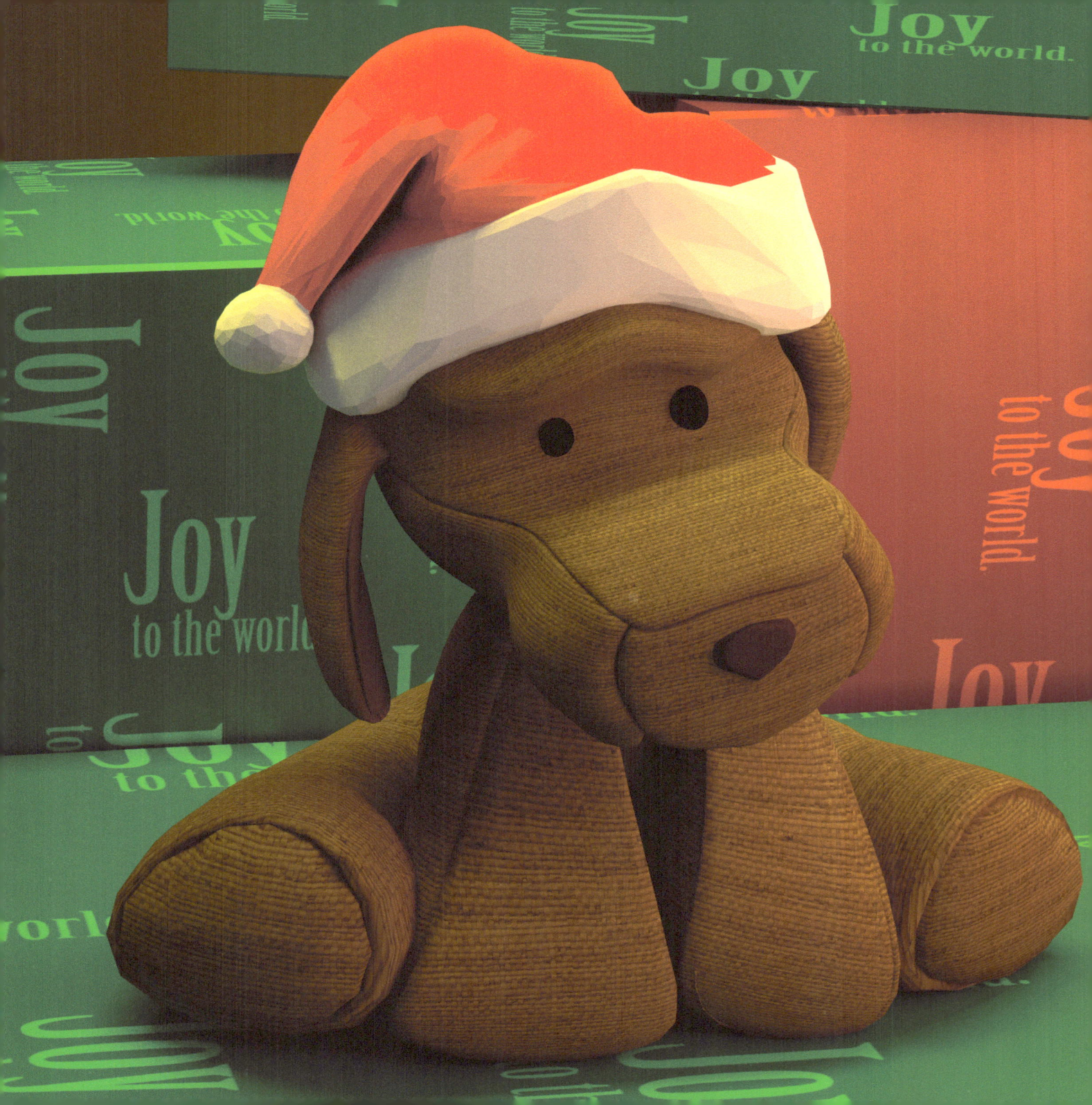

Every day that he's still here,

I have a few less "afraid" tears.

It's not too late to love him.

We weren't sure how Christmas would be.

Would my brother have presents under the tree?

But Christmas was not sad, it was great!

Because he's not dead yet.

Dad sits my brother up on his lap.

He kisses him, tickles him, and makes him laugh.

I worry that he might run out of breath.

When my brother is cute or does something new,

my mom smiles so big. She sees it too.

Then she looks sad and turns away,

but he's not dead yet.

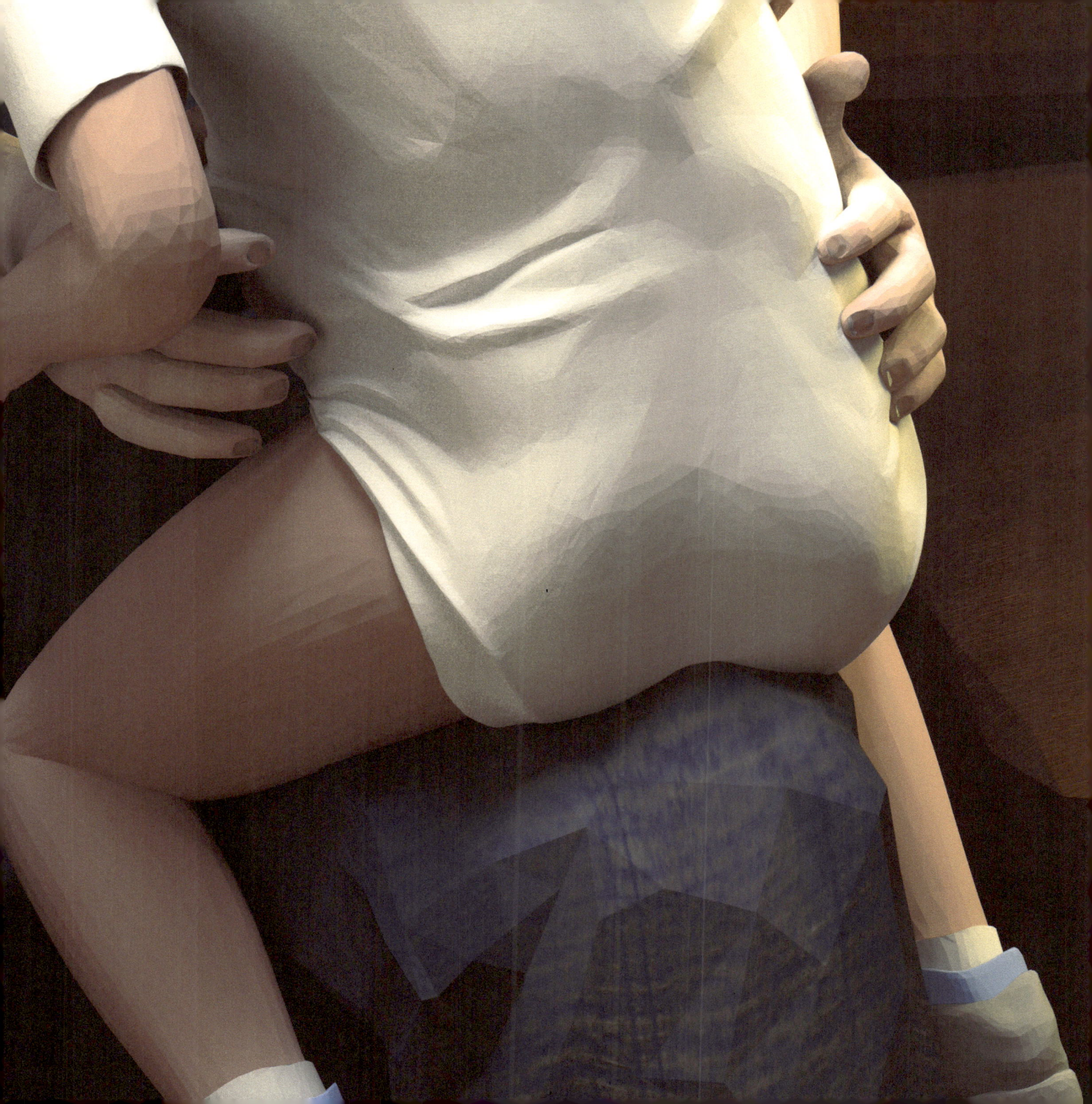

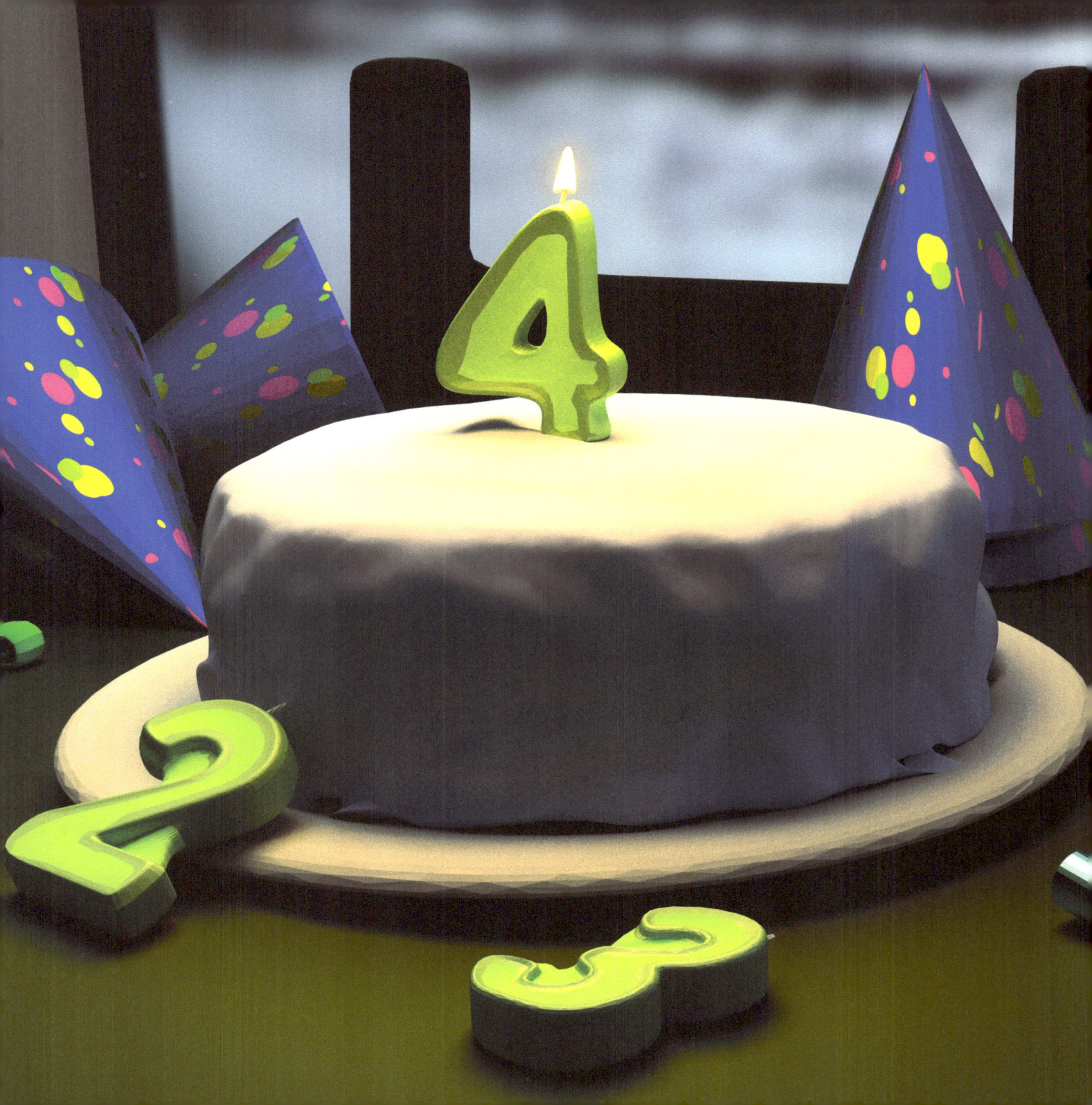

He's not getting weak. He seems pretty strong,

and his hair is growing really long.

Turns out we're having his birthday after all.

People say my brother's brave.

They're all inspired by how we behave,

but he's just him and I'm just me,

and he's not dead yet.

I don't really feel like praying today.

There is nothing left for me to say.

God has heard my prayers before.

My dad told me that my brother is fighting a fight.

There are forces of darkness and forces of light,

and that dragon, cancer, seems to be winning.

Still, he's not dead yet.

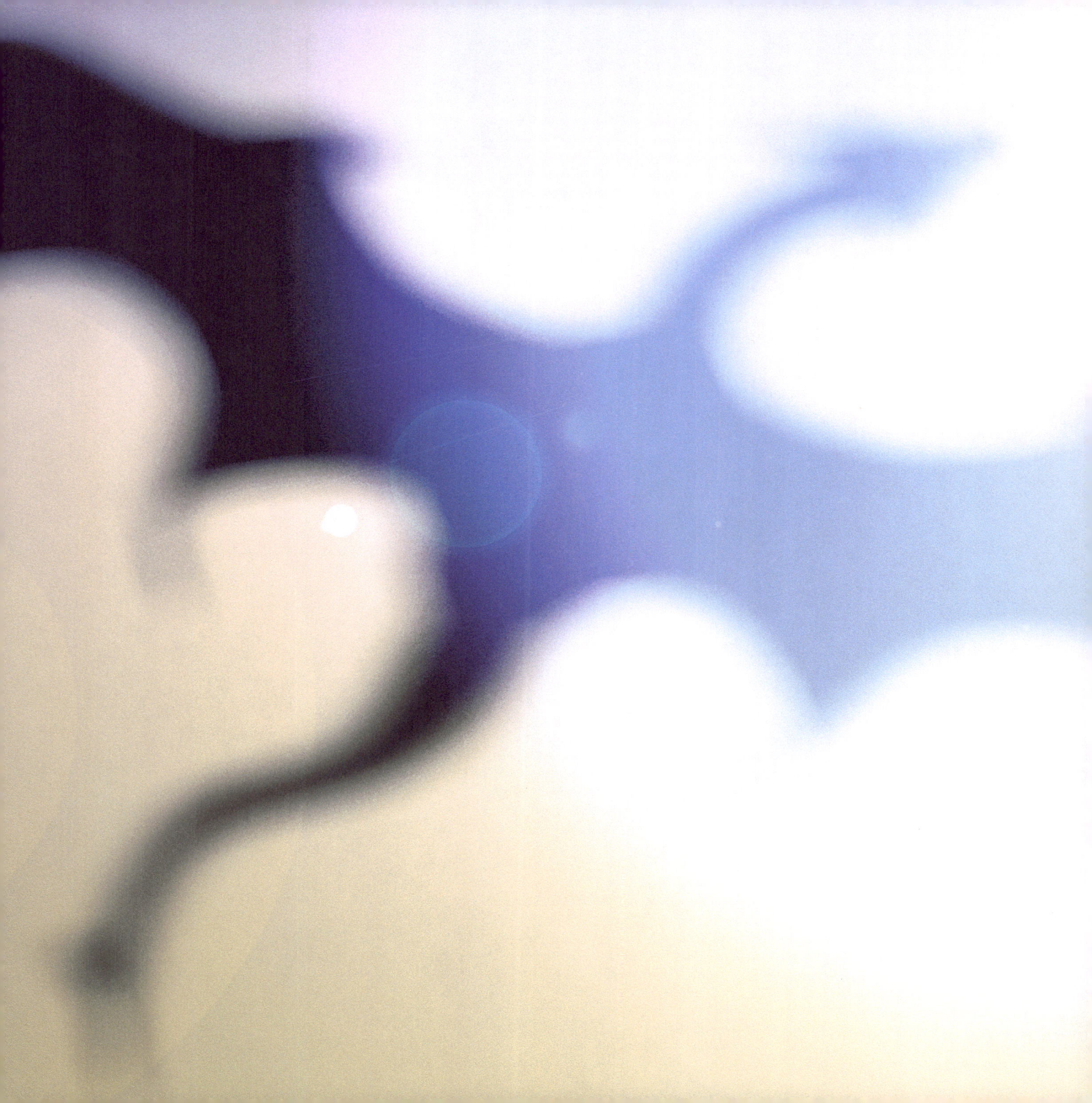

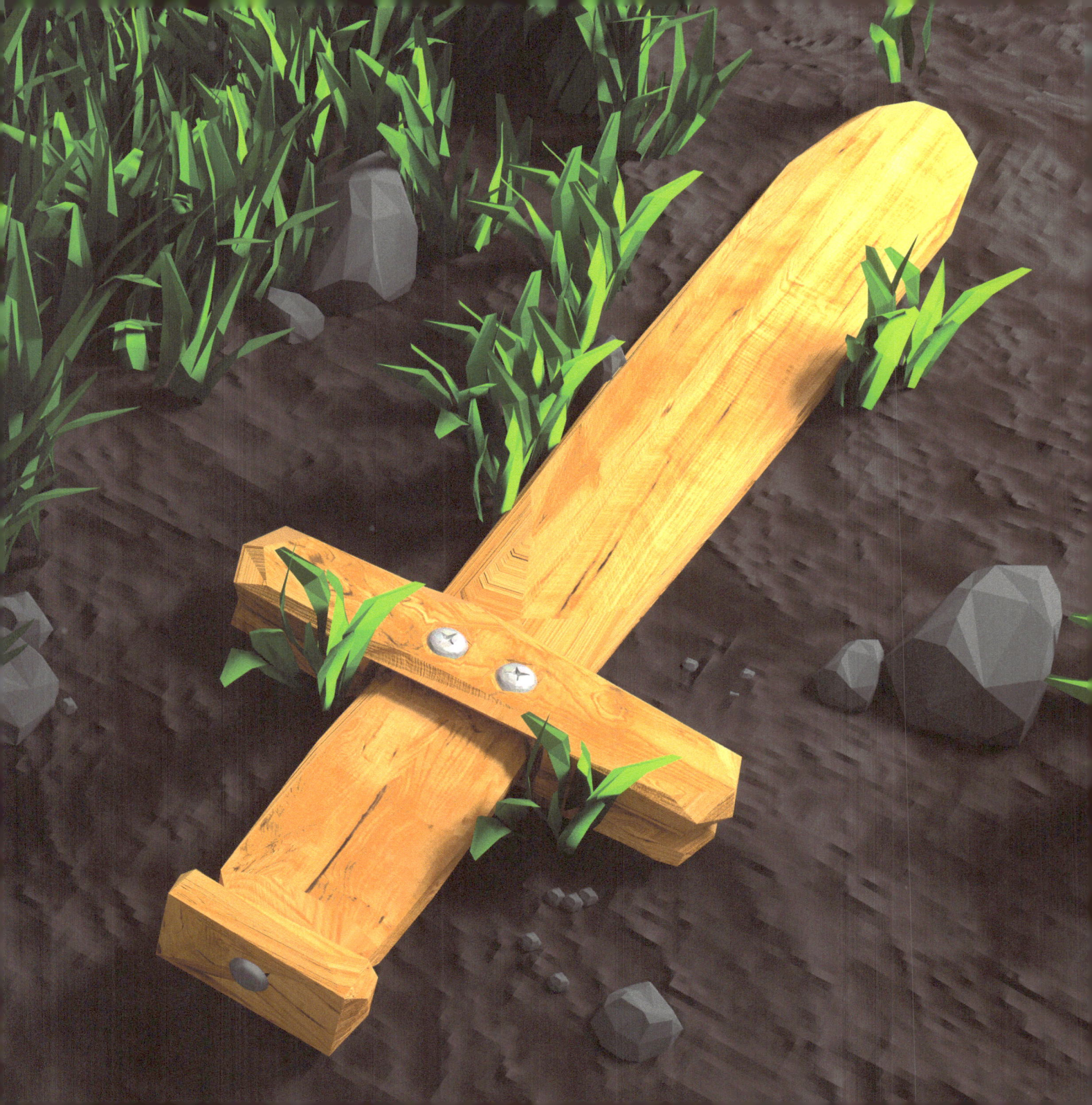

Sometimes it would feel easier to just lie down,

cover my ears and pass on my crown,

but mom called me a king, a warrior, a priest.

I imagine that dragon is big and scary,

but I have a sword that I know how to carry.

Plus, God fights with me, so I'm not afraid.

See, he's not dead yet.

There are too many what ifs for us to think through,

like what if it's April and what if it's June?

No matter when, I will never be ready.

What if my brother grows up even more?

What if we go back to our lives like before?

Maybe what ifs aren't that bad after all,

because he's not dead yet.

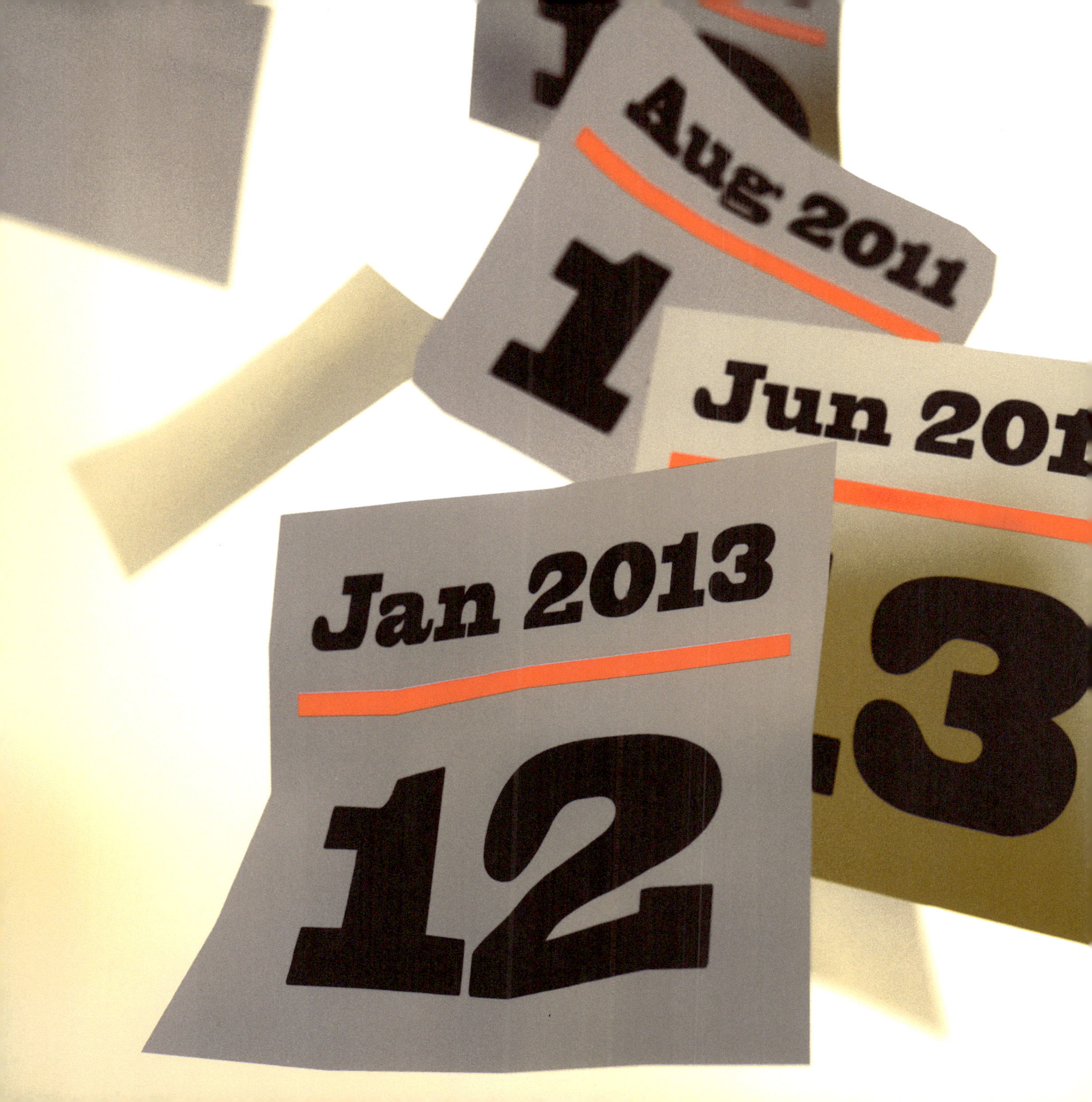

Aug 2011
1
Jan 2013
12

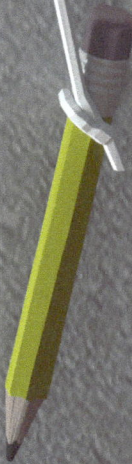

It was only supposed to take weeks or months,

but it's been two years and the end hasn't come.

When will I know if he's past the threat?

The truth is, some days, I forget he's sick.

He's growing hair. He's getting big.

Maybe doctors aren't right every time,

because he's not dead yet.

My mom tells me we're not the only ones in the fight.

People all over the world pray with all their might.

Even though it's hard, we're learning to never give up.

My brother is growing up even more.

It looks like there is a future worth hoping for.

I think there's a chance one day he'll be eighty,

and still not be dead yet.

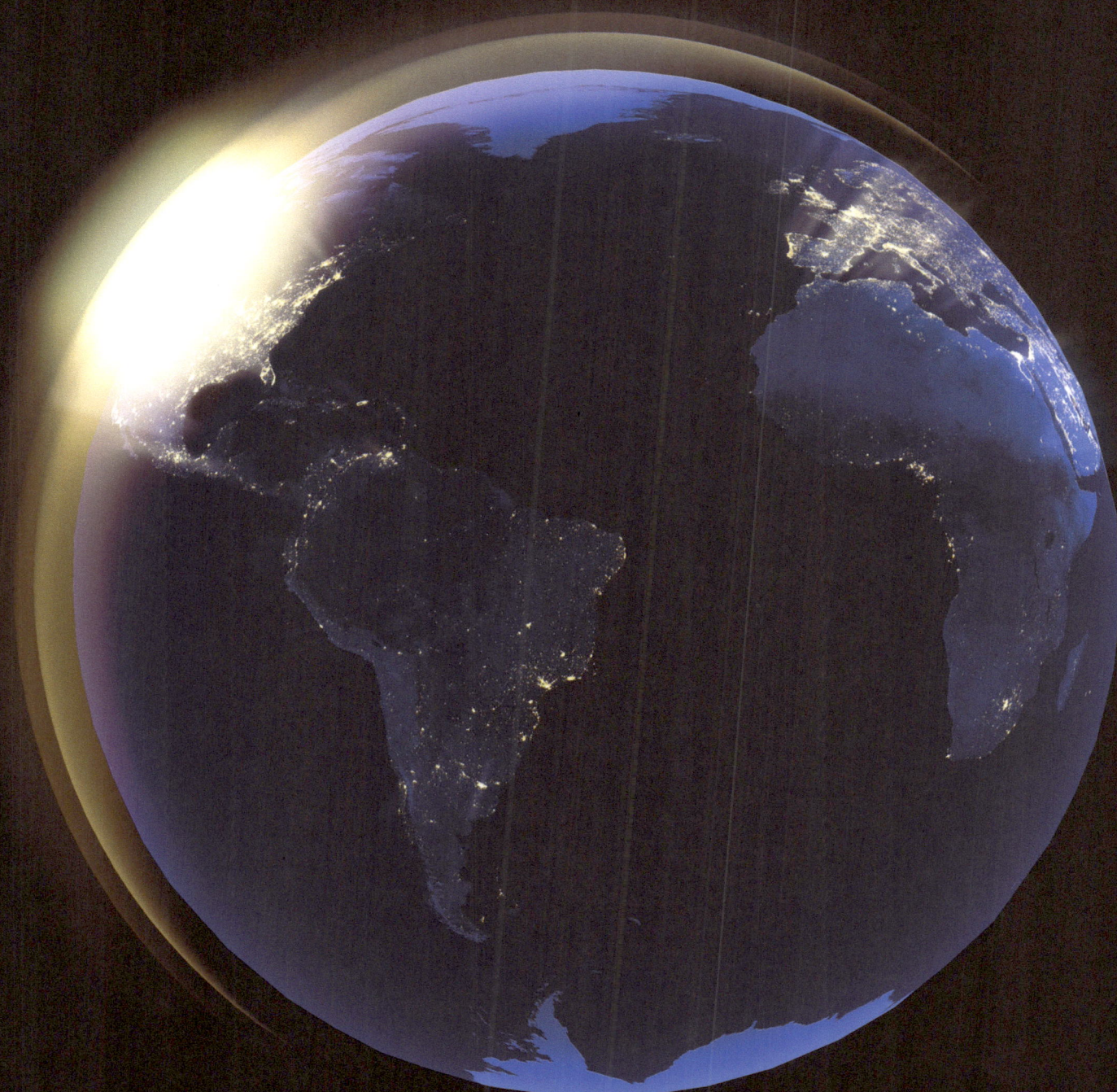

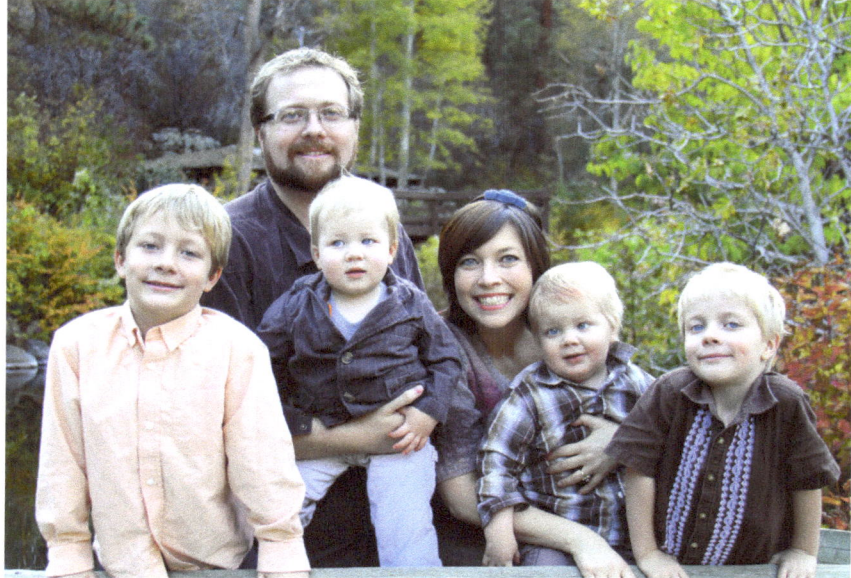

About The Authors

Ryan Green is a programmer and game developer. The proceeds from this book will support his family, as he creates "That Dragon Cancer" a video game that explores sin, sickness and faith. http://www.thatdragoncancer.com Amy Green is a writer, speaker and stand up comedian. Ryan and Amy's greatest aspiration is to raise their four incredible sons (Caleb age 7, Isaac age 5, Joel age 4, and Elijah age 2) to love God without fear.

Joel was diagnosed with an Atypical Teratoid Rhabdoid Tumor (AT/RT) when he was one, and people all over the world began to pray and follow Joel's story on Facebook and on his website http://www.joelevangreen.com Joel had a brain surgery to resect his tumor, 6 weeks of radiation (a treatment usually not given until the age of three but AT/RTs are fast growing and aggressive with a dismal outcome if radiation is not used, and a poor outcome no matter what treatment is used.) Joel received 9 months of the most intense chemotherapy available, and then he had a tumor recurrence.

Three months before Joel turned two he was given a few weeks to four months to live. In the 27 months since then, Joel has had five more tumor recurrences, each one life threatening, and each one treated with palliative treatment, designed to ease symptoms in end-of-life stages of disease. Palliative treatment is not curative.) In October of 2011 Joel was once again expected to die within months, as he had three new tumors. (Two of these tumors ended up dying on palliative iv chemo, the third on radiation.) In November of 2012 Joel's incredible medical team prepared the family once again for Joel's death. His seventh, and most recent, tumor was very large and growing very quickly. Ryan and Amy were told not to expect Joel to have any more long periods of remission. Amy and Ryan Green continue to pray for Joel and are still joined by thousands of people around the world who ask God for more miracles for Joel. The Green family believes Joel will live a long life, and they are dedicated to making the most of every single day that Joel is not dead yet.

Acknowledgements

We want to thank Caleb and Isaac Green whose voices we borrowed, Joel and Elijah Green for being Joel and Elijah Green, and our friends and family for carrying us through the hard seasons. Thank you for encouraging us to share the story of our hearts.

Ryan would like to thank Brock Henderson for his graphic and book design, Josh Larson for his art direction, The Blender Foundation for their excellent and free computer graphics rendering and modeling software at http://blender.org. Sorin at http://render.st for his excellent after hours customer support on their render farm which was used for rendering. http://cgtextures.com for their excellent free texture resource and http://morguefile.com for their free image library. Without the charity of our friends and these organizations, we would not have been able to create this book.)

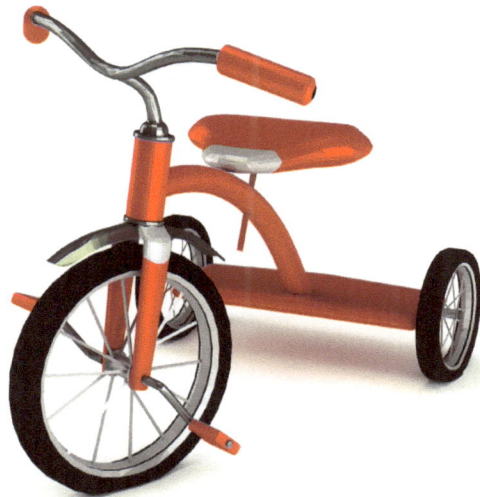